THE POCKET
PEDIATRICIAN

THE POCKET PEDIATRICIAN

650 Tips on Caring for Kids

Michael A. LaCombe, M.D.
Fellow, American College of Physicians

with

William T. Whitney Jr., M.D.
Fellow, American Academy of Pediatrics

ANDREWS AND MCMEEL
A Universal Press Syndicate Company
KANSAS CITY

Library of Congress Cataloging-in-Publication Data

LaCombe, Michael A., 1942–
    The pocket pediatrician : 650 tips on caring for
kids / Michael A. LaCombe.
        p. cm.
    Includes bibliographical references and index.
    ISBN 0-8362-2895-2 (pbk.)
    1. Pediatrics—Popular works. 2. Pediatrics—
Miscellanea.
I. Title.
RJ61.L13   1997
618.92—dc20   96–42122
                                                 CIP

FOR MY KIDS

---

*Mike, Dave, Casey, Caitlin,
Nicole, Thorsten, and Kris*

*Who trained this anxious internist
in primary care pediatrics*

Raising children is difficult enough even as a *physician*-parent. I have often marveled at how well those parents do the job with very little background in medicine. For me, a son's fever of 104°F was frightening, an attack of croup, terrifying. And that morning when my teenager awoke with fever, sore throat, and massive lymph glands, although my intellect whispered "mononucleosis," my emotions screamed "cancer," and I called the doctor.

When *do* you call the doctor, and when can you tough it out? When are fevers, rashes, and runny noses simple rites of passage, and when do they signal an emergency?

Here are tips from a physician-parent who has lived those anxious moments, and who hopes this advice will make those moments less trying for you.

NEWBORNS
AND BABIES

1. Sing lullabies to your baby.

2. Use cornstarch powder, not talcum powder, on your baby.

3. Expect to be depressed during the first week after the birth of your baby. It is common, temporary, and will pass.

4. Diaper rashes get better in three days. Here's what to do:

- Change the diapers frequently.
- Leave the rash exposed to air as much as possible.
- Avoid plastic pants at night.
- Put cornstarch powder on the rash. Remember, never talcum powder.
- Wash the rash only with the mildest of soaps (Basis).

5. If your baby's diaper rash gets blisters or open sores, call your doctor's office that day.

6. Most babies spit up. Smaller feedings help more than burping. The tendency will go away eventually.

7. Babies need hats in winter-
   time.

8. It's impossible to spoil a baby
   during its first three months
   of life.

9. Infants use bumper pads to
   escape, and they will want to
   escape if they can't see out.
   Don't use them.

10. Burping isn't really necessary. Holding is.

11. Maternity leave should last three months at least, and preferably six.

12. Most severe infant diarrhea is caused by viruses. There is now a vaccine available. Ask your doctor.

13. At age six months, a baby can learn to drink from a cup.

14. After age one, vitamin supplements are unnecessary.

15. Never buy a walker for your child. Never.

16. It is normal to breast- or bottle-feed until about eighteen months of age.

17. Sleeping with a bottle of milk or juice can cause severe tooth decay.

18. Get a digital thermometer for your family. They are more accurate and much easier to use.

19. Get the best infant car seat money can buy.

20. For quiet dining at home, the automatic swing is the best invention since candles and wine.

21. The first three months are the toughest. Seriously consider a diaper service.

22. Never microwave your baby's bottle.

23. Humidifiers are better than vaporizers.

24. Accustom your baby to the playpen *before* four months of age.

25. You can make less expensive, more nutritious baby food in a food processor.

26. Treat fever only if over 100°F. And then use Tylenol. Never use aspirin.

27. Fever over 105°F is always a medical emergency.

28. The cardinal signs of
meningitis:

- fever
- stiff neck
- lethargy

But your child, if less than
two years old, need not
exhibit all three.

29. A child can be seriously ill in the first three months of life without having a fever. Treat lethargy, irritability, restlessness, and failure to eat as emergencies.

30. Ask your doctor's office at which time of day telephone consultations are preferred.

31. A baby of twelve pounds at three months of age can relinquish the 2 A.M. feeding.

32. Narrowing of the head from difficult vaginal delivery—called molding—will be gone within the first week of life.

33. The soft spot may close as early as six months or may remain open until eighteen months of age.

34. Children destined to have brown eyes will become so by two months of age. If your baby's eyes are still blue at six months, blue they will remain.

35. The acnelike rash on babies—small red bumps—is just that, neonatal acne. It is caused by maternal hormones, is temporary, and doesn't require treatment.

36. Nipples do not need to be "toughened" before breast-feeding.

37. Soap on nipples will simply dry them out. For lubrication, poke a pinhole in a capsule of vitamin E, squeeze out a few drops, and rub in.

38. To avoid abrasion on a diaper rash, use a blow-dryer set on "low."

39. An undescended testis is not unusual in newborns. But after one year of age, an undescended testis requires surgical correction.

40. For better success with weaning, never let your child hold the bottle, and never let a baby take a bottle to bed.

41. Chicken pox—grouped blisters on a red base—keep erupting for the first five days of the illness. The child is contagious for the first week after the rash starts. The pox won't scar unless the child repeatedly scratches.

42. A fever is an emergency when:

- The temperature is over 105°F.
- The child is listless or unarousable.
- The child has a stiff neck.
- The soft spot is bulging.
- There is a red/purple rash.

43. Rinsing your baby's face with water after feedings will help prevent rash caused by food and stomach acids.

44. When bathing your newborn, keep the water level below the navel until after the cord has fallen off.

45. Fathers: Hold your baby *at least* once a day.

46. If you are breast-feeding, your baby is getting enough:

- if she wants to nurse only about every two hours
- if she seems satisfied after feedings
- if she takes both breasts at each feeding
- and has four or more bowel movements a day
- and wets six or more diapers per day

47. Teething does not cause fever.

48. Teething does not cause diarrhea or diaper rash.

49. Teething rings that will easily chill and hold the cold are favorites with babies.

50. There is enough water in breast milk. Babies do not need extra water.

51. Breast milk does not contain vitamin D or fluoride.

- From age two weeks to twelve years, give fluoride drops.
- Most babies also need vitamin D supplements.

52. If you are bottle-feeding, make sure the formula is iron-fortified.

53. In the first few days of life, it is normal for a baby to lose weight.

54. The average baby will double its birth weight at three to five months.

55. Breast size has no relation-ship to milk production.

56. Immunizations for infants:

- in the first two weeks, hepatitis B
- at two months, first diph- theria-tetanus-pertussis (DTP), oral polio (OPV), hemophilus influenza type B (HIB), hepatitis B
- at four months, second DTP, OPV, HIB
- at six months, third DTP, HIB, and hepatitis B

57. The best owner's manual for parents of newborns is *Dr. Spock's Baby and Child Care* (see bibliography).

58. Most food allergies in infants cause diarrhea, vomiting, hives, or flare-up of eczema.

59. In infants, milk products and eggs are the most common food allergies.

60. Don't give babies whole cow's milk before age one. Use low-fat milk until after age two.

61. When beginning solid foods, start with a rice cereal. It is less allergy-producing. Start at four to six months of age.

62. A pacifier is the best treatment for a colicky baby.

63. It is easier to unspoil a baby than to unspoil an adolescent.

64. Occasional crossing of the eyes is common in babies, but if this occurs most or all of the time, even in the first month, ask your doctor.

65. Delayed weaning from bottle-feeding increases risk of obesity later on.

66. Immunize against whooping cough (pertussis). The risk of brain damage from pertussis vaccine is infinitesimal. The risk of death from whooping cough is far greater.

67. Passive smoking worsens croup.

68. With chest infection, fever, and runny nose, if the wheezing is severe and the breathing difficult and faster than sixty breaths per minute, call your doctor immediately.

69. If your sick child seems to hurt when held or moved, this may be an early symptom of meningitis.

70. Eczema—that red, itchy rash on the cheeks, elbows, and knees—runs in families. Food allergy makes it flare up. Lubricating ointments are the best initial therapy. Try Alpha-Keri bath oil straight from the bottle.

71. Babies who freely use a pacifier don't become thumb-suckers, even when they give up the pacifier at age four months.

72. Babies don't need shoes until they are walking outdoors.

73. *Any* head trauma is an emergency if the child is less than a year old.

74. Most colicky babies do better with lots of cuddling and rocking. Remember, you can't spoil a baby during the first three months of life.

75. By three months of age, your baby should be sleeping in a separate bedroom.

76. By four months of age, most babies will sleep through the night.

77. Most croup gets better on the way to the Emergency Room—when the child is exposed to the moist, cool night air.

78. The thin, watery breast milk produced the first three to four days after birth *is* very nutritious and full of antibodies to help your baby's immunity.

79. There is no medical indication for circumcision in your newborn son. This is entirely your decision, not your doctor's.

80. Notify your pediatrician if your baby does not turn his head to locate sounds by four months of age.

81. Position your sleeping baby on her side or back rather than on her stomach.

82. Make certain your home has smoke detectors.

83. Do not introduce solid foods before four months of age.

84. Between six and ten months of age, expect your baby to crawl, sit, and stand. But remember: some genius babies don't.

85. Put covers on all electrical outlets.

86. Hide all electrical cords.

87. Make certain bathroom doors are closed at all times.

88. Keep houseplants out of reach. Some are deadly poisons.

89. Put gates at the top and bottom of stairs.

90. Store all those cleansers somewhere out of reach, not under the sink.

91. Most birthmarks disappear before the child starts school.

92. Blocked tear ducts are common in babies. The eye tears excessively. There may be swelling and redness. Almost always, this resolves itself without surgery.

93. If your baby is under six months old and is vomiting despite a clear liquid diet, call your doctor.

94. Any baby under six months old with diarrhea warrants a call to the doctor.

95. Warm droplet medication by standing the bottle in warm water for a few minutes. Then your baby will not be shocked by cold drops entering the nose, eyes, or ears.

96. A small swelling in your baby's groin is probably a hernia. Coughing or crying will make it increase in size. Gentle pressure should reduce its size. Consult your doctor.

97. Call your local rescue squad to sign up for a course in Basic Life Support. Learn cardiopulmonary resuscitation (CPR).

98. If you are worried and frightened about your baby, call your doctor.

99. Never leave your baby unattended.

100. The diaper rash that looks like a medical emergency on your firstborn will become routine with her younger brother.

101. Your baby's soft spot will not bulge unless she is crying. If it bulges while she is upright and quiet, call your doctor right away.

102. To remove sand or dirt from your child's eye, hold him under warm, running tap water. You'll need help to hold the eye open.

103. If your child sustains blunt trauma to the eyebrow, expect a handsome black eye.

104. Never put cotton swabs into the ear canal.

105. Always get a second, and even a third, opinion when your child is facing elective major surgery.

106. If your baby cries for several hours and you can't find a cause, call your doctor at once.

107. Unless you relish power games at the dinner table, never spoon-feed your child once he or she can manage a spoon.

108. Let the kids catch you embracing in the kitchen.

109. Don't use Selsun on a baby's
scalp.

110. Jaundice immediately after
birth is quite common and
usually disappears within a
week. But consult with your
doctor anyway.

111. The facial rash of tiny white dots on your newborn baby is called milia. It is never serious and will disappear within three months.

112. Repeated vomiting after meals at about one month of age can result from a congenital narrowing of the bowel called pyloric stenosis —easily curable with minor surgery.

113. Crossed eyes or a lazy eye in your baby beyond three months of age should be brought to the attention of your doctor.

114. You will take more photographs of your firstborn than of all your other children combined.

115. Many children with cerebral palsy are of normal intelligence.

116. Genetics can screen for the carrier state for cystic fibrosis and, by amniocentesis, diagnose cystic fibrosis in the fetus.

117. Babies love classical music. Try Mozart's Twenty-ninth Symphony.

118. Bottle-feeding or nursing your baby in an upright position lessens the frequency of ear infections.

119. Use a suction bulb to remove mucus from your baby's nose. Remember to squeeze the bulb *before* you insert it into the nostril.

120. Never permit your older child to speak for, correct, or fill in sentences for your younger child. This will only worsen stuttering and speech impediments.

121. Learn the Heimlich maneuver for children.

122. Buy flame-retardant clothing and sleepwear only.

123. Never leave an infant lying
on a beanbag chair.

124. Buy a rocking chair. Use it.

125. If, during the last months of your pregnancy, anyone asks how they may help, ask for a frozen meal or two.

126. The umbilical cord stump will fall off sometime between ten and twenty-one days after birth.

127. If your crying baby is inconsolable, check for the open diaper pin, and then for the strand of hair wrapped around a finger, a toe, or the penis.

128. A breast-fed baby can develop diarrhea because of a change in Mother's diet.

129. Double-rinsing all baby clothes and bedding will decrease the possibility of allergic rash from detergents.

130. Your baby should be dressed in one more layer of clothing than you are.

131. The most common error in taking an infant's temperature is failure to shake down the thermometer.

132. Caffeine in the mother's diet may make the breast-fed baby irritable.

133. All babies have two soft spots. The smaller one to the rear closes first.

134. If you are nursing and your baby is colicky, first try eliminating milk products and caffeine from your diet.

135. Strictly limit visitors during the early postpartum period. You will feel you have to entertain, and that will be exhausting for you.

136. Eardrums perforated by infection almost always heal without any residual hearing loss as long as the infection is treated.

137. No one knows the cause of Sudden Infant Death Syndrome. At increased risk are males born in winter, of low birth weight, or of smoking mothers, and babies who are positioned to sleep in the prone position.

138. During the period of breast-
and bottle-feeding, white
patches in your baby's
mouth—thrush, or yeast
infection—can commonly
occur. This is easily treated
by prescription with an oral
antifungal agent.

139. Remember to pin religious artifacts to the baby's clothing. Never use a necklace.

140. Be wary of leaving a jealous older sibling alone with a new baby.

141. When making your own baby food—which is strongly recommended—do not prepare beets, turnips, or carrots, which may be high in nitrates. Better buy commercially prepared jars of these vegetables.

142. Do not use those old-fashioned accordion gates to block stairs and doorways.

143. A toddler's separation anxiety begins at about ten months and is usually gone by the second birthday.

144. Linus's affection for his blanket displays normal childhood behavior.

145. For toddlers, undesirable behavior is best treated with distraction.

146. Remove the dials from your gas stove and reinsert them only when you are cooking.

147. The lid of the toilet, as well as the bathroom door, should always be kept closed when there is a toddler about.

148. It is extremely difficult to tip over a Big Wheel.

149. Remember, in an old house, although the top layer of paint may be lead-free, those underlying layers may not be.

150. Pregnancy after age thirty-five increases the risk of a baby with Down syndrome.

151. Moderate milk intake in your toddler. Milk is filling and may suppress her desire for other necessary foods.

152. The window screen alone will not prevent a child's tragic fall.

153. Don't feed peanut butter to a child under age two.

154. Clean a baby's eyes with a cotton ball dipped in warm water, wiping from the inner to the outer corner of the eye.

155. If your baby has been circumcised, the penis should not be washed until it is healed. Dab petroleum jelly on it to prevent the wound from sticking to the diaper.

156. At eighteen months to three years, the penis foreskin can be retracted for cleaning, but not before then.

157. Sometimes a young girl's labia, the inner lips of her genitals, may fuse due to adhesions. Don't try to separate the labia yourself. See her doctor.

158. Unlike clothes, shoes should not be handed down from one child to another.

159. You can't beat Cheerios for baby's first finger food.

160. If you refinish a crib, make sure the varnish or stain does not give off toxic fumes.

161. Babies sit up at around six months of age.

162. Some babies never crawl. They go immediately from sitting to walking.

163. Infants and small children should always ride in the backseat of a car.

164. You can't speed up your child's development any more than you can speed up his teething. He'll crawl when he's ready.

165. By fifteen months, babies need only one nap a day.

166. Babies need time to be alone too. Don't smother.

TODDLERS AND
YOUNG CHILDREN

167. The reason there are doors on cupboards is for posting children's drawings.

168. Exposure to wind and cold air does not cause pneumonia, nor ear infection.

169. Never give aspirin to a child with fever. Pepto-Bismol contains aspirin.

170. Croup—a tight, barking cough with hoarseness and difficult breathing—is from infection of the vocal cords. Treat with:

- warm mist by humidifier
- a closed bathroom with the hot shower running
- immediate medical attention if breathing is difficult, the muscles between the ribs tug in, your child can't sleep, the child's lips turn blue, or there is no relief from the warm mist after a half hour

Always sleep in the same room with a child with croup.

171. Fever, tugging at the ear, and irritability are signs of ear infection. Antibiotic treatment is required.

172. A child with a cold lasting longer than two weeks should see the doctor.

173. Any child with a strong family history of high cholesterol should have a cholesterol check soon after age two.

174. Measles lasts seven days, and the child is ill. You can't catch measles after the rash is gone.

175. German measles lasts three days, and the illness is mild. Keep the child away from pregnant women.

176. When your child has vomiting and diarrhea from a virus, your job is to prevent dehydration. Use clear liquids for the first day and a bland diet the second day. Pedialyte is a great clear fluid for infants. Use soft drinks with the fizz removed for toddlers and young children.

177. It is normal to get at least six colds a year. Remember, over two hundred different viruses can cause the common cold.

178. The common cold lasts a week with treatment and seven days without. Over-the-counter cold remedies are a waste of money.

179. Immunizations recommended between one and six years:

- twelve months: mumps-measles-rubella (MMR)
- fifteen months: booster hemophilus influenza type B
- eighteen months: fourth DPT shot and third oral polio vaccine (OPV)
- between four and six years: fifth DPT and fourth OPV
- age five: repeat MMR

180. The best reference book for parents regarding illness and disease in children is *Your Child's Health* by Barton D. Schmitt, M.D. (see bibliography).

181. The taste for salt is an acquired taste. Don't let your child acquire it. Don't salt your child's food.

182. Chronic, persistent diarrhea may be caused by apple juice.

183. Never leave a child unattended in a high chair.

184. If you see a worm in your child's bowel movement, save the worm! Correct treatment depends upon it.

185. The only risk from sugar in the diet is tooth decay.

186. Children with egg allergy can get all routine shots except measles and mumps.

187. Passive smoking worsens asthma.

188. Most bronchitis from viruses produces a cough that can last two weeks, but call your doctor if the fever persists beyond three days.

189. The most serious mistake in treating diarrhea is to withhold fluids. This will only worsen the dehydration.

190. Diagnose dehydration by the following:

- no urination for eight hours
- crying without tears
- dry rather than moist mucous membranes
- fever without sweating

191. Persistent fever and nasal discharge with frequent sneezing are more likely from allergy rather than from "a chronic cold."

192. Symptoms of pneumonia:

- rapid, difficult breathing
- frequent cough
- pain with deep breathing
- fever and chills
- abrupt onset of above symptoms after several days of a cold

193. Strep infections require antibiotic treatment for ten full days, no matter how quickly the child's health returns to normal.

194. Hives from food allergy, viruses, or insect bites are best treated initially with Benadryl. You can get it over the counter; follow dosage instructions precisely.

195. The best way to reduce itching from an insect bite is to make a cross on the bite with steady pressure from your fingernail.

196. Impetigo is a streptococcal or staphylococcal infection of the skin. It produces blisters and "honey-crusting," followed by scabs. Oral antibiotics are necessary. Impetigo is very contagious.

197. A child with speech problems at age three or four first needs his or her hearing checked.

198. Turn your hot water heater down to 120°F. Your toddler will be much less likely to scald himself.

199. For sunscreen, use SPF-15 or greater.

200. Even without treatment, most warts will disappear within two to three years.

201. Use changes in diet, not enemas or laxatives, to treat constipation.

202. There is no danger of swallowing the tongue during a convulsion.

203. Consider any head trauma
as an emergency if:
- the trauma is followed by
  a seizure
- the child can't remember
  the accident
- the trauma is followed
  by unconsciousness or
  confusion
- there is a severe headache
- the child begins vomiting
- the child acts confused,
  listless

204. Taking out the tonsils and adenoids will not prevent colds, strep throats, or ear infections.

205. Never compromise about bedtime with a one-year-old.

206. Television violence causes nightmares in children. *Surprised?*

207. Children ages one to ten need ten to twelve hours of sleep per night.

208. Any bite from a household pet that causes swelling, pain, or redness around the puncture wound needs to be seen by the doctor.

209. For bed wetters: There is now an effective, safe bed-wetting alarm to help treat the problem.

210. Stuttering is common between the ages of two and three. Ninety percent of children will outgrow it within a few months.

211. The American Academy of Pediatrics recommends the new chicken pox vaccine—Varivax—for your child.

212. Call your doctor if your child repeatedly complains of pain before or after bowel movements.

213. The following can trigger asthma in your child: cigarette smoke, animal dander, house dust and molds, pollens, cold air, upper respiratory infections, exercise, and, less common, foods and medications.

214. Read to your child regularly.

215. The difference between growing pains and bone cancer is that the pain of bone cancer does not go away. Usually a cancer will cause a swelling and tenderness of the affected bone.

216. If your child has blue lips and difficulty breathing, this is a medical emergency.

217. Cat bites are worse than dog bites. And human bites are worst of all. Seek medical attention.

218. Before you call your doctor's office, take a temperature, count a pulse rate in beats-per-minute, and take a respiratory rate in breaths-per-minute. You can help immensely by taking your child's vital signs.

219. Noncorrosive poisoning is treated by inducing the child to vomit. Keep syrup of ipecac on hand to treat this emergency.

220. The sick child should not be forced to eat. But remember liquids to avoid dehydration.

221. To minimize scarring from scratching itchy rashes, trim your child's fingernails.

222. A rash that does not blanch with pressure may be serious. Press on the rash with the bottom of a clear drinking glass to visualize the effect of pressure.

223. Never break a blister. If it bursts spontaneously, cover it with a bandage and keep it clean and dry.

224. If your child swims in a lake and then appears to be covered with "insect bites," this is swimmer's itch, caused by a bird parasite. Not serious. No treatment necessary. Avoid the lake.

225. A first-degree burn is like a localized severe sunburn. Treat with cold running water, elevation of the affected part of the body, and a clean, dry dressing. Lotions, creams, and topical antibiotics are unnecessary.

226. Chemical and electrical burns require medical attention immediately. Likewise burns on the face.

227. Cold sores near the eye require medical attention. Otherwise, treat with hydrogen peroxide and cover with cold cream.

228. An unexplained cough may be a first symptom of asthma.

229. Notify your doctor if your child does not actively reach for objects by seven months of age.

230. Pediatricians know that telephone reassurance is part of the job. Don't be shy about asking for it.

231. If your child seems too sick to smile, play, walk, or even cry, call a doctor immediately.

232. The DEET in insect repellent can make a child very ill. Spray it on clothing rather than skin.

233. Practice fire drills in your home.

234. Foreign bodies in the eye cannot be "lost" behind the eyeball.

235. Never apply ice or snow to frostbite.

236. If your child drinks caustic solutions, don't induce vomiting. Chemical cleaners, bleaches, gasolines, and furniture polishes are caustic. Give your child milk and get to the emergency room.

237. Any eye injury involving metal chips or shavings requires emergency medical treatment.

238. Blood in the urine is always abnormal.

239. Aspirin causes a bleeding tendency. Don't give it to relieve pain from tissue injury or head trauma.

240. The convenience of bunk beds is outweighed by their potential for trauma. Avoid them.

241. The best disinfectant for cuts and scratches is soap. Iodine, alcohol, and Merthiolate can damage tissues, and they hurt. Hydrogen peroxide is useless.

242. At three years of age, your child can learn the difference between tulip and daffodil, robin and chickadee.

243. Don't worry about fallen arches. It doesn't happen.

244. Almost all childhood infections are caused by viruses. Antibiotics are of no help and can even make matters worse.

245. When your child has a cold and a cough, reserve cough medicines for severe persistent coughs. And get your doctor's advice. Don't waste your money on over-the-counter snake oils.

246. Bacterial infections (e.g., of the ear, lung, or bladder) should improve within forty-eight hours of treatment with antibiotics. If not, call your doctor.

247. Sharing your bed with your child is not recommended.

248. Spare the rod.

249. Use social isolation rather than physical punishment for discipline.

250. Masturbation is perfectly normal.

251. The ideal day-care center should not have television as its focus.

252. Diarrhea with a slight fever is probably from a virus.

253. Diarrhea, slight fever, and pain around the navel or lower right side may well signal appendicitis.

254. Diarrhea, vomiting, and bloody bowel movements constitute an emergency and may be from stoppage in the bowels.

255. If your child has a viral illness with fever and becomes drowsy or difficult to arouse, *always* check with your doctor immediately.

256. Teach your child to be compulsive about hand-washing after trips to the bathroom.

257. The occasional child labeled with "attention deficit disorder" might have petit mal epilepsy.

258. Fever and breathing difficulties are symptoms of pneumonia until proven otherwise.

259. Growing pains:
- are real
- occur *between* the joints rather than *in* the joints
- happen during growth spurts
- come and go
- are not serious
- are best treated with massage and moist heat

260. Scalp wounds always bleed profusely . . . and hemophilia is extremely rare.

261. All parents worry about leukemia. It is extremely rare, and today, eminently curable.

262. Body lice lay eggs at the roots of the hair. Look for them when making a diagnosis.

263. Scabies is quite contagious. The mites usually lay their eggs between the fingers. Look for the rash and the itching to concentrate there. The itching is severe enough to keep the child awake.

264. Remove the stinger from a bee sting by scraping rather than with tweezers.

265. Ignore tantrums. Leave the room. Treat destructiveness with social isolation (time-out periods). Don't call your doctor.

266. Vomiting with runny nose, chest congestion, and mild fever is most likely viral.

267. In Little League, to paraphrase, it is not whether you win or lose, but *whether* you play the game.

268. Pinworms can cause rectal itching and are extremely common and quite contagious. Look for small white worms around the anus, especially at night.

269. Know the difference between poisonous and nonpoisonous houseplants.

270. Don't let your child kiss the dog.

271. Don't let the dog kiss your child.

272. Children learn by example. Wear your seat belt.

273. The first maneuver in treating a drowning victim is mouth-to-mouth resuscitation. Learn CPR.

274. Remember, polio is rare because of immunization, not because the disease has "gone away"

275. Use fluoride toothpastes.

276. Teach your child to floss
daily.

277. A severe sore throat with
fever and trouble swallowing
even saliva constitute a
medical emergency.

278. An asthmatic whose breathing becomes worse and
whose wheezing disappears
needs emergent medical
attention.

279. Avoid fireworks.

280. Keep a fire extinguisher in
the kitchen.

281. Bed-wetting is very rarely psychologically based. In other words, it's not your fault.

282. Bubble baths can cause inflammation of the genital area in girls.

283. Fabric softener sheets used in the clothes dryer are a frequent cause of allergic contact dermatitis.

284. To relieve the itching of chicken pox, give your child a bath in powdered oatmeal (Aveeno brand). Follow directions on the box.

285. Do not use topical cortisone creams on the rash of chicken pox.

286. To relieve the sore nose of a cold, use Chap Stick or petroleum jelly. But if the sore is crusted, this may be impetigo (see tip no. 196).

287. Foods with the artificial sweeteners sorbitol and saccharine can cause diarrhea.

288. Over-the-counter topical cortisone will relieve the severe itching of eczema. Use *ointment* at 1 percent.

289. Children afraid of the dark do much better with a flashlight at the bedside.

290. High fever for three days without an illness, then a drop in the fever and a rash on the fourth day, is roseola —a harmless viral disease.

291. To remove gum from hair, work peanut butter well into the gum, and when you can separate the hair with your fingers, begin to comb out.

292. Avon's Skin-So-Soft is vastly overrated as a mosquito repellent. It works for only twenty minutes. Don't rely on it.

293. Sticky adhesive tape will remove small bits of glass, pieces of shell or coral, and tiny cactus spines from the sole of the foot.

294. Television unsupervised and unregulated by you is largely a negative influence on your child.

295. Calamine lotion is great for the itching of poison ivy. Never use Caladryl.

296. Soak small splinters in warm water first. They will be easier to remove.

297. Praise your child frequently.

298. Two or three drops of rubbing alcohol in the ear will help remove water after swimming.

299. Warm, stale Coca-Cola is still a great rehydrator for the vomiting child.

300. Start the habit of bike helmet with the tricycle.

301. Cook on the back burners of your stove.

302. Keep a phone by the pool.

303. Never move a child suspected of neck injury.

304. At Christmastime, have your children rehabilitate old toys, gift-wrap them, and give them to those children less fortunate.

305. One hour of quality time a day is plenty.

306. Teach your children how to stop, drop, and roll on the ground if clothing catches fire.

307. Children cannot master the mechanics of chewing peanuts until age seven and may choke on them before that age.

308. For scrapes, Telfa pads are nonsticking. Application of an antibiotic ointment will also prevent adherence of gauze to the wound.

309. Never give boiled milk to a child. It is a home remedy more harmful than useful.

310. A child should watch no more than two hours of television per day.

311. An asthmatic child taking theophylline preparations who exhibits nausea and vomiting may be theophylline-toxic.

312. Swollen glands most commonly result from virus infection and, in children, only very rarely from cancer.

313. Reading in poor light does not cause nearsightedness.

314. Take family vacations.

315. Begin swimming lessons as early as possible.

316. You don't have to sleep in a
tent to be a good parent.

317. No child ever willfully
starved himself.

318. Make sure the silk edging of
your child's favorite blanket
is sewn on securely.

319. If at all possible, have an exact duplicate of your child's favorite blanket or toy.

320. Begin early teaching your child respect for the police.

321. Teach your child how to dial 911.

322. A three-year-old should know his or her address.

323. Kissing open wounds promotes infection.

324. As a painkiller, the Band-Aid is second only to a mother's hug.

325. On long car trips, take your child's pillow.

326. Hear both sides.

327. Ampicillin and amoxicillin can give a rash without more serious penicillin allergy.

328. You should tell your adopted child the truth about his or her adoption as soon as he or she is able to understand.

329. A child with a fever will digest fatty foods poorly. Avoid them during a febrile illness.

330. Remember that beets, blackberries, and red food coloring will give the false appearance of blood in the urine.

331. Additives and flavorings in toothpastes can cause rash around the mouth.

332. Berating a child is a form of child abuse.

333. Don't worry about sudden lack of bowel control after successful toilet training. Eliminate stress, and don't make a big deal of it.

334. Decongestants may have a "rebound effect" leading to increased clogging of the nose and ears after the decongestant wears off. Limit their use.

335. Tetracycline may cause teeth staining. It should not be prescribed for children.

336. Foods recommended for a
   nonvomiting, feverish child:
   - toast
   - soup
   - gelatin
   - soft eggs
   - crackers
   - cereal
   - arrowroot cookies

337. Foods not recommended for a nonvomiting, feverish child:
- meat
- sugary snacks
- high-fat items
- fresh fruits and vegetables

338. Roll a fat magazine around a broken arm or leg for an emergency splint. Tie securely without cutting off circulation.

339. Cough syrup may help a coughing child sleep, but it should not be used during the day. The child needs to cough up that mucous.

340. Vaccinations will need to be postponed if your child is running a fever.

341. Never put ointments or butter on a burn.

342. Plant giant sunflower seeds to form a magic outdoor play space.

343. Most children grow out of bowleggedness by four to five years of age.

344. The most common phobia for two-year-olds is fear of dogs.

345. Older preschoolers fear the dark, monsters, desertion, and robbers.

346. Children learn to say no before they learn to say yes.

347. Eighteen-month-old behavior is a harbinger of the terrible twos.

348. Children are at their most difficult halfway between birthdays—at two-and-a-half, three-and-a-half, and so on.

349. Most eighteen-month-olds can pile three or four blocks one on the other and say a few words.

350. Use a rubberized bath mat in the tub to prevent accidents.

351. The best way to avert tantrums is by distraction.

352. If your toddler is always cranky and irritable, he may have a food allergy.

353. Boys lag slightly behind girls in general development.

354. Just as you can't claim full credit for your child's successes, you can't be blamed for all your child's problems.

355. Girls generally begin talking earlier than boys.

356. Crib rocking is a common and normal way for small children to release excess tension.

357. Two-year-olds may fear wind and rainstorms.

358. Putting a harness on your child won't hurt him; being run over by a car will.

359. The terrible twos are really the terrible two-and-a-halfs.

360. Mood swings, sulking, and criticizing parents are traits shared by both terrible twos and teenagers.

361. Even the most active child will be mesmerized and quieted by playing with cups and water in the sink. Buy a step stool.

362. Don't leave your infant alone with your two-year-old.

363. Expecting a two-year-old to share is like expecting an infant to walk—it won't happen.

364. Buy *Goodnight Moon* and make reading it to your child part of your bedtime ritual.

365. The two- to three-year-old's favorite words are "no" and "mine."

366. Three-year-olds commonly have imaginary playmates.

367. Invest in a good stroller and take walks every day.

368. Three-year-olds' hands may have tremors when trying to use fine motor skills. It's normal.

369. Tantrum looming?
- Ask him a question.
- Make a funny face or noise.
- Turn on the radio.
- Distract, distract, distract.

370. Keep a secret supply of inexpensive toys to give your child when you absolutely, positively need some peace and quiet.

371. Many three-year-olds do better with a sitter than with Mother.

372. Stuttering, tripping, blinking, and twitching are very common in three-year-olds.

373. If your child outgrows a nap, you can still have her "pretend nap" so you will both get some rest.

374. Some of the best toys are free: water, sand, big cardboard boxes, playgrounds.

375. As language skills improve, the tantrums will lessen.

376. A good rule of thumb for birthday party guests is this: three for a three-year-old, four for a four-year-old, and so on.

377. Make up a story and ask your child to tell you how it will end.

378. Clowns scare most small children.

379. You can't expect good table manners before the age of five or six.

380. Allow your child to use whichever hand she wants, right or left.

381. Little boys worry that their penises will be cut off or fall off. Reassure them.

382. Precocious children, such as those who read at an early age, often slow down as they get older and even out with the other children.

383. Four-year-olds' most common words are "why," "hate," and "please." Swearing is common.

384. Four is the age for running away from home and for locking oneself in the bathroom.

385. Young children delight in real stories of what their parents did—both good and bad—when they were young.

386. *Where the Wild Things Are* was undoubtedly written about a four-year-old.

387. Four-year-olds are fascinated by urinating and defecating.

388. A four-year-old can be verbally and physically aggressive and violent toward a much older sibling.

389. Children always fuss and act up when Mother is on the telephone. Try to save long calls for nap time or when they are at day care.

390. Whispering can often work better than shouting. Your child has to quiet down and concentrate in order to hear you.

391. Four-year-olds are both afraid of and fascinated by fire. Hide the matches and lighters.

392. Ignoring swearing is possible. This behavior will pass.

393. Your child's first two-wheel bike should be small enough so his feet can touch the ground when it is upright.

394. When your child uses a word incorrectly, don't correct her. Rather, repeat what she said, using the word correctly.

395. Play the favorites game. Ask your youngster, "What is your favorite . . . (dessert, animal, food, color, toy, etc.)?"

396. Keep preschoolers' birthday parties short, about one-and-a-half hours.

397. Don't push your preschoolers to read.

398. Girls should be five and boys should be five-and-a-half before starting kindergarten.

399. Learn some knock-knock jokes to amuse your preschoolers.

400. Play Twenty Questions during long car rides or waiting times.

401. Don't be surprised at how violent your children's made-up stories can be. Even children who aren't allowed to watch TV tell violent stories. It's developmental.

402. It's okay to feel a temporary dislike for your child. Just don't let him or her know.

403. Four- and five-year-olds frequently lie. It passes.

404. Imaginary friends are perfectly normal.

405. Children whine more to Mom than to Dad.

406. It's a good idea for twins to be in separate classrooms when they start school.

407. Eight-year-olds are accident prone. Buy kneepads and a helmet.

408. Eight is a good year to start an allowance.

409. Seven-year-olds frequently cling.

LATE CHILDHOOD
AND ADOLESCENCE

410. A child with infectious mononucleosis must avoid contact sports for six to eight weeks.

411. Children with asthma or cystic fibrosis should have flu shots.

412. No one can diagnose a strep throat by physical examination. The only way to tell is with a throat culture or Quick-strep test.

413. Improperly treated strep throats are a cause of rheumatic heart disease.

414. For painful breasts during adolescence, use over-the-counter ibuprofen as directed (Motrin, Advil, Nuprin).

415. Athletic teenage girls with breast pain most likely need better breast support. Get a good jogging bra, the best you can afford.

416. Pinkeye is extremely contagious. Expect every child in the household to get it. Seek treatment with topical antibiotics if the eyelids are crusted together in the morning.

417. Begin acne treatment with:
- strict cleanliness to rid the face of oils
- a drying soap in the morning (Pernox, Fostex)
- 5–10 percent benzoyl peroxide lotion at bedtime

418. There is no evidence that foods such as chocolate, strawberries, or tomatoes cause adolescent acne.

419. For severe acne, unresponsive to home remedies, ask your doctor about antibiotic treatment or treatment with Accutane.

420. The child with infectious
mononucleosis and fever
is at the most contagious
stage.

421. Scarlet fever—rough, dry,
sunburned skin following a
sore throat and fever—needs
treatment with penicillin-
like drugs.

422. Bladder infections are not uncommon in young girls. The signs and symptoms:

- burning on urination
- increased frequency of urination
- urinating in small amounts
- fever and belly pain

Treatment with antibiotics is required.

423. To prevent bladder infections, teach your daughter to wipe front to back, not back to front.

424. Never embarrass your child.

425. Immunizations between ten and sixteen years:

- ten to twelve years: mumps-measles-rubella, hepatitis B
- fourteen to sixteen years: tetanus-diphtheria booster

426. Most bed-wetting occurs in boys. Three to 5 percent of boys still wet the bed at twelve years of age, but most stop in adolescence.

427. To combat foot odor:

- wash daily
- powder the feet and shoes with an over-the-counter antifungal powder
- never wear the same shoes two days in a row
- change socks at least twice a day and always wear cotton socks

428. To combat dandruff:

- shampoo more often, not less
- start with a mild shampoo
- if no success, switch to Selsun Blue
- get some sun exposure

429. The best way to get your child to wear a seat belt is for you to use one. If you don't buckle up, she won't.

430. Passive cigarette smoking increases the risk of sinus infection, sore throat, pneumonia, bronchitis, influenza, ear infection, and school absenteeism.

431. Sudden severe pain in the groin should not be passed off as "a hernia." Twisting of the testis in the scrotum needs surgical treatment within eight hours.

432. Earplugs and cotton plugs will not prevent ear infections. Don't use them.

433. Blackhead "poppers" are perfectly okay for removing blackheads.

434. Rash with cracking between the toes, burning skin on the feet, and unpleasant odor are symptoms of athlete's foot. Treat as you would foot odor (see tip no. 427).

435. Boils on the skin are common, especially in athletic adolescents who frequent gyms and locker rooms. Treat by washing the entire body with an antibacterial soap. Showers are better than baths, since the infection is less likely to be spread to other parts of the body.

436. The best treatment for dry, cracked hands is lanolinized hydrous wool fat. Your pharmacist can get it for you. No prescription necessary.

437. The best home remedy for a bee sting is to rub the sting with a cotton ball soaked in meat tenderizer solution.

438. To treat jock itch, buy over-the-counter Tinactin or Micatin spray. Wash and dry the area thoroughly twice a day, then apply the spray. The rule is to apply the medication for a week *after* the rash has gone.

439. Never make your child ashamed of you.

440. Most processed meats contain fat, salt, nitrates, and poor quality meat. Be choosy about what you feed your children.

441. For head and body lice, get Nix. It contains the antilice shampoo and a fine-toothed comb for removing the nits or eggs from body hair. You don't need to shave the hair to cure lice.

442. Poison ivy lasts two weeks.

443. When do the stitches come out?

- face——three to four days
- scalp, chest, arms, and hands——one week
- legs, feet, backs, palms, and soles——ten to fourteen days

444. Ringworm—an oval-shaped pink patch with scaly borders and a clear center—is caused by a fungus infection often contracted from household pets. Apply over-the-counter Tinactin cream or Lotrimin cream twice a day until one week after the rash is gone.

445. Common among all children of divorce is their assumption of responsibility for it. Reassure them, often, that they are not to blame.

446. Reassure children of divorce that it is not incumbent on them to bring their parents back together.

447. Should you get an infestation of scabies in your household, you do not need to wash every stitch of bedding. Scabies cannot live outside the human host for longer than three days.

448. Children with shingles can spread chicken pox to others.

449. Breast cancer is extremely rare in teenagers. The finding of a lump under the nipple is common in boys.

450. Ibuprofen is excellent treatment for menstrual cramps. Get it over-the-counter as Motrin, Advil, or Nuprin.

451. A cold washcloth applied anywhere to the face, head, or neck will not stop a nose-bleed.

452. A cut needs stitches if the edges are separated, or if the cut is longer than half an inch (or a quarter of an inch on the face).

453. For sunburn of the eyelids, apply tea bags soaked in cool water.

454. Any wild-animal bite, including that of a squirrel or raccoon, needs to be seen by a doctor immediately.

455. Treat pizza burn—the scalding of the roof of the mouth by hot foods—with ice. Immediately put an ice cube in the child's mouth.

456. A teaspoon of sugar is a great cure for hiccups.

457. Onset of first menses occurs around age twelve, and the periods for the first year or two will be irregular and infrequent, as a norm.

458. Most adolescents become ashamed of their parents for a time. That shame usually disappears by the time college tuition payments come due.

459. An abscess is a local collection of pus. Never drain it yourself. Don't pinch it or lance it.

460. The pain of appendicitis usually begins in the pit of the stomach and then moves to localize in the right lower abdomen.

461. A child with appendicitis will not want to eat.

462. Abdominal pain made worse by walking or by coughing or sneezing requires immediate medical attention.

463. The cardinal symptoms of diabetes mellitus are increased urination, increased thirst, and increased appetite. Weight loss and fatigue develop. Don't ignore these symptoms in your child.

464. Remember that one cause for missed menstrual periods is pregnancy.

465. Teach your daughter how to change a flat tire.

466. Sudden loss of interest in schoolwork, sports, and friends, a depressed mood, and preoccupation with death are symptoms of suicide risk in an adolescent.

467. Skunks, raccoons, bats, and foxes carry rabies. Squirrels sometimes do. Chipmunks, rabbits, mice, and rats do not.

468. On hot summer days, bring ice water to the Little League games.

469. High fever without sweating is a symptom of heat stroke and requires emergent treatment.

470. Tell your budding athlete never to use salt tablets.

471. Treat sprains with RICE: **R**est, **I**ce, **C**ompression, **E**levation.

472. Any cut on the eyeball or eyelid should be treated by a doctor.

473. A puncture wound is always potentially serious, especially when through a sneaker, or when caused by a dirty nail. Err on the side of talking to your physician.

474. Treat the loss of a permanent tooth as a medical emergency. Get your child to the dentist immediately and bring along the tooth in a glass of *milk*.

475. Skipping breakfast is never a good idea.

476. Your child should get a second mumps-measles-rubella vaccine at about twelve years of age.

477. Your rules are not negotiable.

478. Video games are preferable to television. Neither is preferable to reading.

479. When allowing R-rated movies into your home, think about who will be watching them.

480. Dyslexia can be subtle, sometimes not diagnosed until college age. Think about it when encountering school difficulties with your child.

481. Sore throat, fever, lethargy, and markedly swollen glands manifest infectious mononucleosis.

482. Let your child overhear you praising her.

483. A headache on one side of the head associated with nausea and aversion to light could be migraine. Remember, migraine runs in families.

484. Frequent hives, together with a family history, warrant a doctor's attention.

485. Warts on the soles of the feet can be quite painful and should be treated. Freezing them with liquid nitrogen is virtually painless, and curative.

486. Scoliosis—curvature of the spine—is not uncommon in adolescent girls. Easily visible if looked for, it should be brought to the attention of your doctor. Make sure your school has a screening program.

487. Equip your home with fire extinguishers.

488. Teach your child to be wary of strangers. Teach this often.

489. You will frequently wish you could send your fourteen-year-old off to reform school. That is a normal emotion.

490. Unprotected sun exposure increases risk of skin cancer later in life.

491. Most heart murmurs in teenagers are innocent murmurs and should not lead to restriction of physical activity.

492. Teenagers who depend only on condoms for birth control risk a 20 percent chance of pregnancy in the first year of sexual exposure.

493. Parental love and strict parenting are not mutually exclusive.

494. Genital herpes produces sores on the cervix, vagina, or penis with discharge, painful urination, and swollen glands in the groin.

495. Teenagers need at least eight hours of sleep each night.

496. The teenage girl with anorexia commonly has low self-esteem, is a perfectionist, obsessive, and preoccupied with body image.

497. Teenagers suspected of anorexia *require* professional help.

498. Teenage girls with severe migraine should not use birth control pills.

499. Twenty-five percent of teenage girls are sexually abused before eighteen years of age.

500. Never apply ice to an injured scrotum.

501. Teenage boys should be taught testicular self-examination for cancer.

502. Weight loss, fatigue, inattention, and irritability all can be symptoms of substance abuse.

503. It is normal for teenagers to take risks. It is the parents' task to see that the risks don't result in injury.

504. Motor vehicle accidents are the leading cause of death in teenagers. Think about it.

505. Birth control pills do not protect against sexually transmitted diseases. Safe sex means condoms or abstinence.

506. By age nineteen, over half of all adolescents have had sexual intercourse.

507. Tattooing, pierced ears, and nose rings increase one's risk of HIV infection and of hepatitis B and C.

508. If you suspect your child is a suicide risk, remove guns from the home, then get professional help.

509. Hypercriticism teaches rebellion.

510. You cannot catch AIDS by sharing gym equipment, showers, or swimming pools.

511. Most adolescent girls commonly have one breast larger than the other.

512. The normal menstrual cycle is twenty to thirty-six days, with the average at twenty-eight days.

513. Participation in team sports is a great confidence-builder for the adolescent girl.

514. The adolescent girl without sexual exposure does not need a Pap smear.

515. Adolescent girls should be taught breast self-examination.

516. Three-quarters of sexually active teenagers do not practice contraception.

517. Healthy teenagers do not need flu shots.

518. It is common for teenage boys to experience temporary breast enlargement. This will disappear within two years and does not require surgery.

519. Teenage girls with ovulatory pain (rather than appendicitis) do not have fever, nausea and vomiting, or loss of appetite.

520. Chest pain in an adolescent is rarely serious.

521. Teenagers at risk for sudden death from heart disease usually have a family history of same.

522. Rock music and rock concerts are risk factors for permanent hearing loss.

523. Jewelry containing nickel is a frequent cause of contact rash.

524. Masturbation does not cause acne.

525. After exposure to HIV infection, it can take three to six months to develop a positive blood test.

526. Douching (with Coca-Cola or with anything else) will not prevent pregnancy, syphilis, or AIDS.

527. Never use a tampon for longer than six hours.

528. It is normal for early adolescents to be attracted to members of the same sex.

529. Any facial boil needs to be examined by a physician.

530. Chewable Tums will decrease the pain of canker sores.

531. The normal frequency for bowel movements ranges from three times a day to three times a week.

532. A piece of dental floss under the edge of a toenail will help prevent ingrown toenails.

533. Children are no different from adults—their tension headaches are best relieved with massage.

534. A bath in finely powdered oatmeal (Aveeno brand) will relieve the itching of hives.

535. Muscle cramps in your adolescent athlete best respond to massage. Teenagers still love touching, however otherwise the reaction.

536. TV addiction produces a bored, whiny child always demanding to be entertained.

537. The government of Iceland has banned television on Thursdays in the interests of promoting reading and family life.

538. When disciplining your child, do not withdraw your love.

539. The nature of the rules is less important than your consistency in enforcing them.

540. Don't forget tetanus boosters. Forty percent of people who get tetanus die from it.

541. If you were subject to the raging hormonal fluxes of adolescence, you would have periods of temporary insanity too.

542. If you choose not to force your child to finish dinner, don't let him fill up on junk food later.

543. Catch and release.

544. Assign chores beginning at
age five.

545. A weekly allowance is a
good idea. Find out what
the neighborhood kids are
getting.

546. Every child living in your home should have a bedtime or a curfew.

547. If you have more than one child, plan to spend individual time with each.

548. Sandboxes are a great reservoir for pinworms.

549. A child over three who swallows a penny, a nickel, or a dime can usually pass it without difficulty.

550. A child who throws candy or nuts in the air, catching them in his mouth, risks blockage of an air passage.

551. A child who wants a pet should care for and feed it. It is not your job.

552. When your first child reaches puberty, that is a good time to order Call Waiting.

553. A separate phone line is not a right of adolescence. It is a privilege.

554. Don't joust at windmills. At any one time have no more than five rules, but stick to them.

555. You will know what your teenager is at risk for when you know what his friends are up to.

556. Teenagers are no different from anyone else. They have great difficulty in separating wants from needs.

557. Have your teenager learn CPR. It will give him a sense of power and of responsibility.

558. Learn how to use a telescope with your child.

559. Teach your child her way around the heavens at night.

560. Permit attacks of silliness. They are a necessary part of growing up.

561. To be a good parent, you needn't attend every single school event. Attend the ones important to your child.

562. Fathers: Tell your daughter—often—how beautiful she is.

563. Start a support group for mothers of fifteen-year-old daughters.

564. When parenting teenagers, it is perfectly normal to harbor evil thoughts.

565. The emotion of love and the impulse to lock teenagers away are not mutually exclusive.

566. You will never understand a teenager's preference for music. Give it up.

567. The more you try to be your teenager's buddy, the more difficult it will be to be his parent.

568. Leave the task of spoiling your children to their grandparents.

569. *The Brady Bunch* was fiction.

570. If at all possible, try not to employ your children for the summer.

571. Places every kid should visit: Boston's Museum of Science, the San Diego Zoo, the Grand Canyon, the Smithsonian's Air and Space Museum, your state's parks, the National Portrait Gallery in Washington, D.C., the

Cleveland Zoo and Rain Forest, Toronto's Science Center, Rochester, New York's Strassenburg Planetarium, Montreal's Aquarium, North Carolina's Outer Beaches, and Maine's Acadia National Park.

572. Things every kid should do: Fly a kite, swim in a lake, play in the ocean, ride a bike, build a sand castle, sleep in a tent, run a lemonade stand, go ice-skating, pick strawberries, bake a cake, plant a tree, play miniature golf, attend a

small-town parade, see fireworks on the Fourth of July,
have a chat with Santa
Claus, roll down a grassy
hill, pick wildflowers, go
tobogganing, jump in a pile
of leaves, host a child from
a foreign land, and give gifts
as well as receive them.

573. Most things are better by morning.

574. A real flashlight makes a great present.

575. For the kid who seems to have everything: books.

576. Teach your child how to use the public library.

577. The preteenager has not been invented who can handle all the sexuality on MTV.

578. If you think when your child graduates from high school your parenting days are over, just wait a few months.

579. For children, cross-country skiing is as much fun as downhill and far less expensive.

580. The best thing a father can do for his children is love their mother.

581. Children will respect their mother if their father does.

582. Have your son or daughter spend a day at work with you.

583. When checking into a hotel, have the kids carry the luggage. But do order ice cream from room service.

584. Don't be surprised if the motel pool is the biggest kid-pleaser on your family vacation.

585. Teach your children the whys and hows of tipping for service.

586. "Sir" and "Ma'am" are graceful Southern habits every child should learn.

587. Encourage your child to participate in at least one sport each year.

588. Children do not require brand-new athletic equipment until they are fully grown.

589. The PTA is not a must, but visiting with your child's teacher is.

590. Kitchen magnets were invented to hold family photographs to the refrigerator door.

591. Expect stirrings of adolescence at eleven, the beginning of the breaking away
from Mom and Dad.

592. Three shots of hepatitis B
vaccine are required for
eleven-year-olds.

593. Ages eleven and thirteen are
bumpy years, but twelve is
easygoing.

594. Gifted children should not skip grades. It is more important to be placed according to emotional maturity.

595. Ten is a happy, well-adjusted age, the calm before the storm. Enjoy it while you can.

596. Adultlike table manners generally occur at around ages ten to eleven.

597. Eleven-year-olds are very critical and argumentative with Mom.

598. Your child will become a bottomless pit for food at eleven or twelve—good news for parents of finicky eaters.

599. Shoplifting is more prevalent among eleven- and twleve-year-olds than with any other age group.

600. Girls become interested in boys long before boys become interested in girls.

601. Children disappear into their rooms at thirteen. They'll reappear in a year or so. Don't worry. Feed them when they emerge.

602. If your young teen has frequent embarrassing erections, have him try wearing an athletic supporter during school.

603. Young teens prefer a lock on their bedroom door. This is dangerous in case of fire. Don't allow it.

604. A great, inexpensive gift for your teen is a full-length door mirror.

605. Consider buying workout equipment, a punching bag, or a gym membership for your teenager; he can take out his tension and aggression there instead of on you.

606. Parents are stupid and embarrassing to a fourteen-year-old, but we seem to grow smarter in the ensuing ten years.

607. Children learn violence in the home, not from TV.

608. Don't pry or interrogate. Take a long car ride with your teen and one or more of her friends and eavesdrop.

609. If you blow up, yell, and scream, simply apologize later. You are normal.

610. Try not to ridicule or accuse.

611. Compliment your teen on those things she does right.

612. Although teens still value family, they shouldn't have to attend every family function. And you can allow them to leave early.

613. Write out house rules and stick them on the refrigerator.

614. Before interfering in a teen's minor school troubles, ask whether your help is wanted.

615. Hang up a list of bathroom rules:

Hang up your towel.
Wipe up spilled water.
Change the toilet paper if
you use it up.

616. Make it a rule that you only
wash the clothes that make
it to the hamper or laundry
room.

617. Hands and feet grow first, then arms and legs. Can you wonder why teens are so clumsy?

618. Don't laugh when your son asks for a razor when he has only a few facial hairs.

619. Remind your teen that a pierced belly button takes up to a year to heal. Do they want that hassle?

620. Catch your children doing something good.

621. Brothers and sisters should have the same set of rules.

622. If your child has a long-range project, help her break it down into steps and make a schedule.

623. If your house is full of reading material, your children will be readers.

624. Don't pay money for good or improved grades, but do reward them.

625. Get involved in your child's school activities and watch his or her grades improve.

626. "Don't judge a book by its cover" is never truer than during the teen years.

627. Encourage your teenager to entertain friends at home.

628. Meet with the guidance counselor at least once a year.

629. Beware of colleges that accept anyone who is able to pay.

630. Establish rules for using the Internet. The kids should never:

- give out their full name, address, or phone number
- share their password with a friend
- access X-rated adult sites or newsgroups

631. Watch your athletic daughter for eating disorders.

632. If your teen dislikes organized sports, encourage bicycling or in-line skating or swimming.

633. Driver's education is a must.

634. Make sure you review what to do if your young driver has a car accident.

635. Honor-roll students and those who have completed driver's education classes often get discounts on car insurance rates.

636. Teenagers need at least seven to nine hours of sleep a night.

637. Exercise helps relieve depression and stress in teens.

638. Worry about suicide if your teenager starts giving away his most treasured possessions.

639. Potbellies on otherwise slim children could signal a vitamin D deficiency.

640. A *painless* red sore on the penis can be a sign of syphilis.

641. The Job Corps and Americorps are wonderful opportunities for the non-college-bound senior.

642. Venereal warts are transmitted sexually and are more contagious than other warts.

643. How to pick up a teenager's room for him or her:

- Line large trash can with trash bag.
- Throw everything on floor into trash bag.
- Repeat with as many trash bags as is necessary.
- Put trash bags in cellar.
- This rarely needs to be done more than two or three times.

It gets results.

644. Signs of Legg-Perthes disease:

- limping
- pain in leg
- pain and stiffness in hip and thigh

645. Hiccup cures:

- Hold one's breath to the count of ten.
- Breathe into a paper bag.
- Quickly drink a glass of water.
- Eat dry bread.
- Eat a teaspoon of sugar.

646. During your child's teen years, preserve your sanity with a sense of humor. It's the only way.

647. Excessive earwax can be caused by exposure to dust- and debris-filled air.

648. Unpasteurized milk, cheese, and butter harbor the brucella bacteria. Don't serve them.

649. Weight loss with bad-smelling, large stools, gas, and diarrhea can mean your child is abusing laxatives or mineral oil to lose weight.

650. If your teen wants to lose weight, suggest swimming, bicycling, skiing, and jogging—these activities burn the most calories.

Dr. Michael LaCombe has practiced general internal medicine for over twenty years in rural Maine, is Director Emeritus of the American Board of Internal Medicine, a Regent of the American College of Physicians, and associate editor of the *Annals of Internal Medicine* and the *American Journal of Medicine*.

BIBLIOGRAPHY

Dr. Spock's Baby and Child Care, by Benjamin Spock, M.D., and Michael B. Rothenberg, M.D., 6th Ed., 1992, Pocket Books, New York.

Instructions for Pediatric Patients, by Barton D. Schmitt, M.D., 1992, W. B. Saunders Co., Philadelphia.

Baby and Child A to Z Medical Handbook, by Miriam Stoppard, M.D., 1992, The Body Press/Perigee Books, New York.

Your Child's Health, by Barton D. Schmitt, M.D., 1991, Bantam Books, New York.

Caring for your Baby and Young Child Birth to Age Five, by Steven Shelov, M.D., 1993, Bantam Books, New York.

Complete Baby and Child Care, by Miriam Stoppard, M.D., 1995, Dorling Kindersley, London.

INDEX

TOPIC   **ITEM NUMBER**

A

abscess. 459
accidents 350, 407
acne 417, 418, 419, 433
adolescence 515, 541, 591
adoption. 328
aggression 605
AIDS. 510, 526
allergies. 58, 59, 186, 191, 194, 283, 352
allowances 408, 545
Americorps 641
amniocentesis 116
anorexia 496, 497
antibiotics 193, 244, 327
appendicitis 253, 460, 461
arthritis. 644
aspirin 169, 239
asthma 187, 213, 228, 278, 311, 411
athlete's foot 434
attention deficit disorder. 257

B

bacterial infection 246
bed-wetting 209, 281, 426
bee sting 264, 437
behavior 347, 348, 359, 360, 362, 363, 365, 371,
                              379, 384, 388, 389, 601, 603
birthday party 376, 396
birthmarks. 91
bites 208, 217, 224, 454, 467
blackheads. 433
bladder infections 422, 423
blankets. 144

blinking.. 372
blister 223
body piercing.................................. 619
boils...................................... 435, 529
books...................................... 57, 180
bowel movements 531
bowel movements: bloody 254
bowleggedness................................. 343
breast-feeding 16, 36, 46, 50, 51, 55, 78, 128, 132, 134
breasts 511, 515, 518
breasts: painful............................ 414, 415
bronchitis 188
bumper pads 9
burns 225, 226, 341, 455
burping 10

c

caffeine 132
cancer 312
cancer: bone 215
cancer: breast 449
cancer: skin 490
cancer: testis 501
canker sores.................................. 530
car safety 163
car seat 19
cereal.. 61
cerebral palsy................................ 115
chicken pox 41, 284, 285, 448
chicken pox vaccine........................... 211
choking 307, 550
cholesterol................................... 173
circumcision 79, 155
clinging...................................... 409
clothes....................................... 130

cold sores. 227
colds 172, 177, 178, 191, 192, 245
colic 74, 134
constipation. 201, 212
convulsion 202, 203
cornstarch 2, 4
cough. 228, 245
cough syrup. 245, 339
cramps: muscle 535
crawling. 84
crib rocking. 356
croup 67, 77, 170
crying 127
cup. 13
cuts 241, 260, 308, 323, 452, 472, 473
cystic fibrosis 116, 411

D

dandruff. 428
day care 251
decongestants 334
DEET. 232
dehydration 190
depression 3, 135, 466, 508
development 229, 242, 322, 457, 458, 486, 489
diabetes 463
diaper rash 4, 5, 38, 48, 100
diarrhea 12, 48, 94, 128, 176, 182, 189, 252, 254, 287
discipline 145, 248, 249, 265, 297, 326, 332, 477,
                                                489, 538, 539, 554, 581
disinfectant 241
divorce. 445, 446
doctor. 98, 106, 218, 230
doctor: telephone calls. 30
dogs 270, 271

douching 526
Down syndrome. 150
driving 633, 634
drops 95
drowning 273
dyslexia 480

E

earplugs. 432
ears 104, 136, 168, 171, 197, 204, 246,
                            298, 430, 432, 507, 522
earwax 647
eating disorders 631, 649
eating habits 598
eczema. 70, 288
epilepsy 257
erections 602
exercise 632, 637, 650
eye color 34
eyes 92, 102, 103, 113, 154, 227, 234, 237, 313, 472
eyes: crossing. 64

F

fatigue 481, 502
feeding: bottle 52
feedings 16, 17, 22, 25, 31, 37, 58, 59, 60, 61, 83,
                    107, 118, 132, 138, 141, 151, 176, 181, 220,
                    307, 317, 329, 440, 475, 542
feet 243, 293, 427, 434, 485, 532
fever 26, 27, 28, 42, 47, 169, 171, 192, 255,
                    258, 266, 277, 290, 329, 469, 481
finger food. 159
fire extinguishers. 487
fishing 543
flu shots. 411, 517

fluoride 51
friends 627
frostbite 235
fun 571, 572

G

games 395
gifted children 594
gifts 574, 575, 604
grades 624, 625, 635
growing pains 259
gum 291

H

handedness 380
hats 7
head 32, 73
head trauma 203, 239
headache 203, 483, 533
hearing 80
heart disease 521
heart murmurs 491
heat stroke 469
hemophilia 260
hepatitis 507
hepatitis B vaccine 592
hernia 96, 431
herpes: genital 494
hiccups 456, 645
high chair 183
HIV 507, 525
hives 194, 484, 534
homosexuality 528
house rules 613, 615, 616, 621, 630
humidifiers 23

I

illness 29, 68, 69, 93, 216, 220, 231, 573
imaginary playmates 366, 404
immunizations 56, 66, 179, 211, 274, 425,
                                                          476, 540
impetigo 196
infection 648
ingrown toenail 532
insect bites 194, 195, 292

J

jaundice 110
Job Corps 641
jock itch 438
jokes 399

L

labia 157
language skills 375
leukemia 261
lice 262, 441
lips: blue 216
lying 403

M

manners 585, 586
masturbation 250, 524
maternity leave 11
measles 174, 175
meningitis 28, 69
menstruation 457, 464, 512
migraine 483, 498
milestones 161, 162, 164, 349, 353, 355,
milk 60, 309
money 545
mononucleosis 410, 420, 481

movies 479
mucus 119, 191, 266, 286
music 117, 522, 566

N

napping 165, 373
nearsightedness 313
neck 303
newborns 1, 21, 44
nightmares 206
nosebleed 451

O

opposite sex 600

P

pacifier 62, 71
pain: abdominal 462
pain: chest 520
pain: ovulatory 519
painkillers 324, 414, 450
paint: lead 149
Pap smear 514
parenting 314, 316, 319, 320, 328, 424,
              439, 445, 446, 482, 493, 509, 544, 547,
              555, 558, 559, 560, 562, 563, 567,
              569, 578, 580, 582, 590
peanut butter 153
peanuts 307, 550
penis foreskin 156
pennies 549
Pepto-Bismol 169
pets 551
phobia 344, 345, 357, 378, 381, 391
pinkeye 416
pinworms 268, 548

playpen 24
pneumonia........................... 168, 192, 258, 430
poison 236, 269
poison ivy.................................. 295, 442
poisoning................................... 219
polio 274
pool 302, 584
precocious children............................. 382
pregnancy 150, 492

R

rabies... 467
rash 35, 43, 70, 111, 129, 138, 174, 221,
                222, 224, 263, 282, 283, 284, 290, 295,
                327, 331, 434, 438, 447, 484, 523
reading................................. 214, 397, 623
ringworm.................................... 444
roseola.................................... 290

S

safety....... 85–90, 97, 99, 121, 122, 123, 139, 140, 142, 146,
            149, 153, 170, 198, 233, 240, 256, 269, 272,
            279, 280, 300, 301, 306, 318, 321, 322, 429,
            465, 468, 487, 503, 504, 550, 557
salt... 181
scabies 263, 447
scalp 109
scarlet fever 421
school........................... 561, 589, 625, 628, 629
scoliosis....................................... 486
scrotum....................................... 500
seat belts 429
separation anxiety 143
sex.......................... 499, 505, 506, 514, 516, 577

shingles 448
shoes 72, 158
shoplifting 599
SIDS 137
sitting 84
skiing 579
skin 436
sleep 75, 76, 81, 205, 207, 209, 240,
                          247, 289, 495, 546, 636
smoke detectors 82
smoking 187, 430
soft spot 33, 101, 133
sore throat 277
speech 120, 197
spitting up 6
splint 338
splinters 296
spoiling 8, 63, 570
sports 267, 410, 468, 470, 491, 513, 579, 587, 588
sprains 471
standing 84
stitches 443, 452
strep infection 193, 204
strep throat 412, 413
stuttering 210, 372
sugar 185
suicide 638
sunburn 453, 490
sunscreen 199
surgery 105
swallowing 277
swearing 383, 392
swimming 315
swing 20

swollen glands 312
syphilis 640

T

table manners 596
talcum powder..................................... 2
tampons... 527
tantrums............................. 265, 351, 369, 375
tattooing 507
teenagers................. 495, 496, 555, 563, 564, 566, 567
teeth.. 275, 276, 474
teething 47, 48, 49
telephone...................................... 552, 553
television 206, 251, 294, 310, 478, 536, 537, 577
tension... 605
testis 431, 501
testis: undescended 39
tetracycline 335
thermometer 18, 131, 218
thrush 138
toilet training 333
tonsils 204
toxic fumes 160
toys 374
tremors 368
trips.. 325
twins 406
two-wheel bike..................................... 393

U

umbilical cord 126
urination: painful 494
urine: blood in.................................. 238, 330

V

vacations 571, 583, 584
vaccinations.................................... 340
vaporizers 23
venereal warts 642
violence 401, 607
virus 175, 176, 244, 252, 255, 312
vitamins.................................... 14, 51
vitamin D deficiency 639
vomiting..................... 93, 112, 176, 203, 236, 254,
                              266, 299, 311

W

walkers 15
warts 200, 485
weaning....................................... 40, 65
weight 53, 54
weight loss.................................. 463, 502
whining....................................... 405
work.................................... 570, 582
worms 184